✎ Doctor Guide Book Series

Wound Care
General Principles

By
Kenneth Wright in consultation with Lyla Reichart

A special thanks to the selected members of The Physicians Association for Patient Education, WOCN and ET nurses, who assisted in developing this book from suggestions and their own printed educational material.

Also a special recognition to the Association for the Advancement of Wound Care (AAWC) and the Canadian Association of Wound Care (CAWC)

ISBN 978-1-896616-11-7
© 2016 Mediscript Communications Inc.

Wound care. Wounds. Self help wounds Chronic wounds First edition. All rights reserved.

The publisher, Mediscript Communications Inc., acknowledges the financial support of the Government of Canada through the Book Publishing Industry Development Program (BPIDP) for our publishing activities.

Printed in Canada

TABLE OF CONTENTS

Introduction

Wound care is a broad subject encompassing many different types of wounds and many different medical specialists. The aim of this book is to provide a bridge between the medical specialists and the patient, caregiver, family members and health care workers.

As a reader, you want a basic understanding of this health condition and pointers on who is at risk, self care procedures and treatment options, as well as an understanding of the tests and treatments and a realistic expectation of healing.

The two broad categories of wounds are acute and chronic. Acute wounds are usually traumatic, such as a cut, scrape or other skin injury. They generally heal quickly if simple hygiene and maintenance procedures are followed.

Chronic wounds can be instigated by some kind of trauma, but the driving force behind their development is skin that has become vulnerable because of a wide variety of factors, such as old age, diabetes, high blood venous pressure, poor nutrition, fragile skin or incontinence.

A chronic wound involves an underlying problem; consequently, it can take a long time to heal, requiring an enormous amount of time and care-giving. In order to provide effective care, one must understand the principles of wound care – ultimately, prevention is of primary importance.

It is much better to prevent a wound from occurring than to try to heal a wound, especially a chronic wound. Prevention involves a mix of common sense and understanding how wounds develop and faithfully following wound prevention guidelines.

If and when a wound does develop, or you spot the tell-tale signs or symptoms, early intervention is critical. Inform the medical staff immediately if you suspect the patient has a problem – the timeline is crucial.

The true nature of wound care is both an art and a science. The art lies in the health professional's skill and chosen procedure in applying the preferred regimen for managing the wound and the surrounding skin.

The science refers to the health professional's knowledge and understanding f the disease process coupled with the correct treatment.

This combination of art and science, together with all the variables of products and procedures available, means that facilities, physicians and nurses will have many different approaches. One approach is not necessarily better than the other; rather, there is a great deal of variety in treatment and many different journeys towards the same healthy outcome – the healing or prevention of wounds.

0309WC2009

INTRODUCING THE SKIN

In order to understand wounds it is important to understand the anatomy of the skin and to appreciate the blood circulatory system which supplies the skin with nutrients and oxygen.

The following diagram shows the various components of the skin

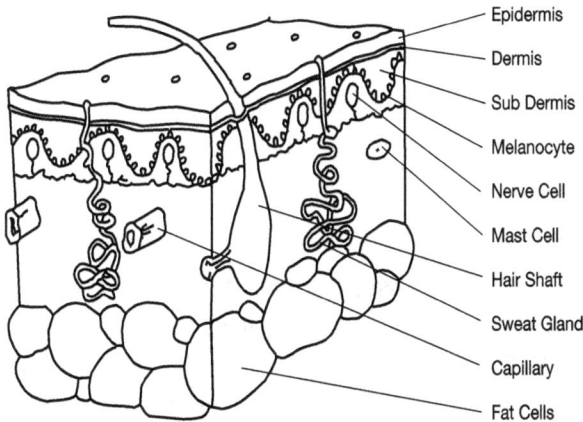

Labels:
- Epidermis
- Dermis
- Sub Dermis
- Melanocyte
- Nerve Cell
- Mast Cell
- Hair Shaft
- Sweat Gland
- Capillary
- Fat Cells

Cross Section of Skin

The skin is actually classified as an organ like the heart or lungs and has many functions such as sensory, regulates body temperature, protecting the inner body and excreting certain body fluids.

The skin is made up of separate layers that function as a single unit. There are two distinct layers, the epidermis and dermis, that lie above a layer of subcutaneous fatty tissue, called the hypodermis.

The epidermis and dermis contain five structural networks

including collagen fibres, elastic fibres, small blood vessels (capillaries), nerve fibres and lymphatic vessels.

The capillaries carry the blood supply oxygen and nutrients to the cells of the dermis by way of a process called capillary filtration where fluids pass through the capillary walls. It is important to understand this because sometimes when the blood circulatory system is compromised - e.g. through diabetes, or venous disease - healing of wounds is made more difficult because oxygen and nutrients are having difficulty reaching the wound area.

Every square inch of skin contains 15 feet of blood vessels.

The skin's lymphatic system helps remove waste products such as excess proteins and fluids from the dermis.

Melanocytes are responsible for the colour of skin by producing the pigment melanin.

The subcutaneous tissue or hypodermis contains layers of loose connective tissue that contains a lot of blood vessels, lymph vessels and nerves. The function of this layer is to insulate the body, absorb shock to the skeletal system and help the skin move easily over underlying structures. In men the subcutaneous tissue can be 15%-20% of total weight, in women it can be 20% - 25%.

A contributing factor to many wounds is the fragile skin that develops in elderly people.

There is a 1% decrease each year in the collagen levels in the dermis of the skin, causing a thinning of the outer layer of the skin (the epidermis and dermis). Collagen provides the skin's tensile strength so loss of it can contribute to wrinkling. Also, elastin fibers in the dermis of the skin provide the skin's elasticity. Loss of this elastin contributes to the skin's tendency to sag and wrinkle.

Aside from the obvious change in the skin's appearance, the so-called "fragile" skin is a major contributing factor to the development of pressure ulcers and other skin problems.

Here are the changes to the skin due to aging.

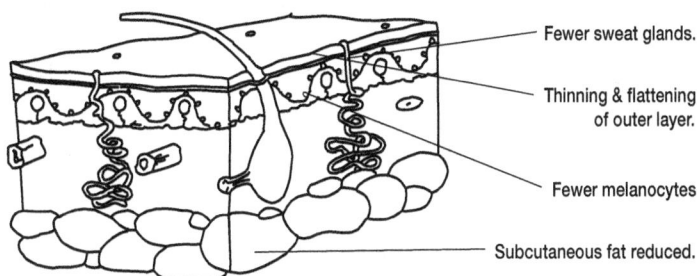

Fewer sweat glands.

Thinning & flattening of outer layer.

Fewer melanocytes

Subcutaneous fat reduced.

Diagram of aging skin

Increased dryness of the skin

Over time, the eccrine glands decrease and the sweat glands produce less sweat. This collectively contributes to drier skin. Hydration of the skin is a fine balance for the elderly person; under- and over-hydration of the skin are fundamental causes of unhealthy skin. Over-hydration can be caused by perspiration or even exudates seeping from a wound.

Less blood circulation

As the skin's dermis thins, fewer blood vessels are available leading to a decreased blood supply. This means there are fewer nutrients, oxygen and other components vital for the healing process being circulated within the body.

Slowing epidermis cell replacement

Renewed cells are replaced at a slower rate which has implications for vital skin health and for any healing process that needs to take place.

Sensory decline

Due to a variety of reasons such as nerve damage or loss and decreased blood circulation, there is a gradual decrease in sensation to pressure and light touch. This is particularly prevalent in people with diabetes where this loss of sensation (also known as neuropathy) is worsened by high blood sugar.

Less immunity to infection

There is a loss of Langerhans cells which are responsible for the development of the bacteria-fighting defense mechanisms of the epidermis in order to counteract skin infections.

Loss of hair and pigment of the skin

There is a decrease in the melanocytes (the pigment-producing cells) which can lead to the loss of melanin and cause graying of the hair and reduced hair growth.

Loss of skin's full, healthy look

The subcutaneous fat on the hands, face, shins, waist (in men) and thighs (in women) tends to atrophy over time, leading to sagging and folds in the skin.

In conclusion, we know wounds are caused by a breakdown of the skin and this is usually obvious. However the skin usually provides signs and symptoms prior to wound formation so it is important to be systematic, vigilant and to know what you are looking for to prevent a wound developing. The following chart provides a comprehensive overview of all the possible relevant observations that can help in being proactive towards either prevention of the wound or early treatment.

WOUND HEALING

Any break in the skin is considered a wound. Skin damage in wounds varies widely, from a superficial cut in the epithelium to a deep pressure ulcer wound that can penetrate as deep as the bone.

The rate of wound recovery varies according to the extent and type of damage incurred and other factors such as patient nutrition, hydration and blood circulation. However although these recovery rates will vary, the healing process is much the same in all cases.

Types of wound healing

A wound can be classified by the way it closes.

Primary intention

This involves the skin's outer layer (epidermis) growing closed, this is called re – epithelialization. Cells grow in from the margins of the wound and out from the epithelial cells lining the hair follicles and sweat glands.

Examples of these wounds are superficial wounds that only involve the epidermis with no loss of tissue such as a first degree burn. A surgical incision also heals by primary intention because it has well – approximated edges (edges that can be pulled together to meet neatly).

Secondary intention

These wounds have some sort of tissue loss with edges that cannot be easily approximated, pressure ulcers and serious burns are examples.

During healing, the wounds fill with granulation tissue; then a scar forms and re - epithelialization occurs, primarily from the wound edges. These wounds take longer to heal, result in scarring and can have a high rate of complications compared to the primary intention healing category.

Tertiary intention

These wounds are intentionally kept open to allow edema or infection to resolve or to allow for the removal of exudate. They are eventually closed with sutures, staples or adhesive skin closures.

Phases of wound healing

Whatever the cause of a wound, the healing process is always the same and consists of four phases: hemostasis, inflammation, proliferation and maturation. It is worth understanding that the healing process rarely proceeds in this strict order and there can be considerable overlap between the four processes.

Hemostasis (stopping the bleeding)

Immediately after an injury, the body releases biochemicals that begin the process of cleaning and healing the wound.

Another word for hemostasis is vasoconstriction, meaning the walls of blood vessels contract, reducing the flow of blood to the injury and minimizing blood loss.

There is then a process involving many other biochemicals from the blood to prevent further blood loss with the eventual formation of a blood clot.

Inflammation

This is a defense mechanism and an important component of the healing process in which the wound is cleaned and rebuilding begins. During this process serous fluid which transports critical amounts of cells and protein accumulate in tissue around the wound causing edema or swelling, which causes the damaged tissue to appear swollen, red and warm to touch.

Various types of white blood cells spearhead the defensive function of removing bacteria and other contaminants. Growth factors within the fluids now aid in the process of granulation and rebuilding the epithelium. The bottom line of this phase is to prevent infection.

Proliferation (growth)

This is the rebuilding phase where the wound is filled with connective tissue, the wound edges contract and the wound is covered with new epithelium (epithelialization).

All wounds go through the proliferation phase but it can take much longer with wounds with extensive tissue loss.

This phase also involves the regeneration of blood vessels and the formation of granulation tissue. As the wound bed forms, this area dons a red "beefy", granular appearance, giving the appearance of progress in healing, although it can bleed quite easily.

Maturation

This is marked by the shrinking and strengthening of the scar. This is a gradual phase of healing and, depending upon the individual, can continue for months or even years, after the wound has closed.

Factors that can affect wound healing

If you are a caregiver you can appreciate the importance of comprehensive quality care for patients in ensuring a healthy outcome. The most important factors include the following:

Nutrition

Proper nutrition is one of the most important factors in wound healing; malnutrition is, unfortunately, one of the most common findings among patients with wounds. Protein is crucial for wounds to heal properly and it is often recommended that a person double the recommended allowance for protein. A patient who lacks protein usually suffers from a slow healing wound. The reason for the need for protein is for the formation of collagen for the proliferation phase of healing.

Another important benchmark to evaluate nutritional health is to measure the amount of albumin in the body. Albumin is a protein manufactured by the liver and it performs many vital functions such as ensuring optimum transportation of nutrients and oxygen to the wound area.

Moisture/Humidity

Maintaining a moist wound environment has been proven to assist the healing process, providing the following advantages:

a) Prevents tissue dehydration, helping to stop the formation of a scab or dry crust (eschar) on the top of the wound. This eschar can hinder the migration of newly-formed skin cells (the technical name is epithelial cells) to the surface of the skin. These new cells can only move through the thin watery liquid within the wound– that liquid is called the serous exudate;

b) increases the growth of new blood vessels;

c) assists in the interaction of the growth factors in the target cells

d) reduces the chances of infection

e) is associated with less pain.

Oxygenation

Wound healing depends upon adequate oxygen for a variety of reasons including helping fibroblasts stimulate collagen synthesis and assisting leucocytes destroy bacteria and thereby prevent infection. There are many possible causes of inadequate oxygen including poor arterial flow, pressure, COPD and peripheral vascular disease.

Debridement

This is the technical term for removing any blood clots, scabs or dry crust on the wound. This can be achieved by the following four methods:

a) Surgical – removing tissue using a scalpel or scissors;

b) Mechanical – referring to a range of techniques like wet-to-dry dressings, wound irrigation or whirlpool or foot soaks;

c) Enymatic – using collagens

d) Autolytic – using dressings such as hydrogels which enhance the body's own enzymes.

Debridement is needed to ensure a moist wound environment in order for the wound to heal.

Exudates

Secretions of fluid are produced by the inflammatory response of the wound. This exudate actively promotes healing through its nutrients and provides an ideal fluid for the new skin cells to move or migrate to the new skin "building sites."

Temperature

Wounds should be kept covered to maintain optimum physiological temperatures. Cleansing agents should be used at body temperature.

Infection

Infection slows down the healing process and extends the inflammatory response. Infections must be eliminated as soon as possible; the physician will use creams, ointments or antibiotics to clear up this problem.

You should try to be vigilant and look for the early signs of infection such as redness, heat, pain, odour, discolouration of granular tissue, and drainage around the wound area.

Smoking cigarettes

It is worth mentioning this as a stand alone negative factor for many reasons. The major factor relates to carbon monoxide a major gaseous component of smoke that binds to the hemoglobin in red blood cells thereby reducing the levels of vital oxygen being transported by the blood to the wound area.

Nicotine is a powerful vasoconstrictor that narrows peripheral blood vessels thereby reducing the amount of oxygen to the wound site.

Finally, lung tissue damaged by smoke does not function as well as it should , resulting in decreased oxygen levels.

There are many more reasons to quit smoking related to wound healing and there are now many effective treatments / nicotine substitutes available that can help patients quit.

Intrinsic factors

Advancing age, combined with a slower metabolic process and associated reduced collagen and poor circulation can impede the healing process.

A range of disease processes can adversely affect the ability of the wound to heal; these include anemia, arteriosclerosis, cancer, cardiovascular disorders, diabetes, immune disorders, inflammatory diseases, liver problems, rheumatoid arthritis and uremia.

Psychological factors like stress and anxiety can also affect the immune system and can disturb sleep which is important for the healing of wounds.

In conclusion the main point in the healing process is to remove all adverse influences. Nature has set a healing time for each type of wound and that healing will only occur if conditions are favourable.

ACUTE & CHRONIC WOUNDS

The difference between an acute wound and chronic wound is based on certain characteristics. You cannot always differentiate the types by length of time to heal because there is not a set time frame before an acute wound becomes a chronic wound. Here is a chart differentiating the differences

ACUTE	CHRONIC
A new wound	Usually develop over time
Occurs suddenly	Healing is slow
Heals by primary intention	Heals by secondary intention
Healing usually progress in a predictable manner	Typical examples are pressure ulcers, diabetic foot ulcers
Typical examples are trauma accidents, first aid type wounds and surgical wounds	Often there is an underlying disease

ACUTE WOUNDS

Acute wounds are often regarded as superficial and a first aid approach is the order of the day, knowing that the powerful ally is the body's natural ability to heal itself.

Some acute wounds as a result of a gunshot or a car accident can be massive and traumatic. However, in the less intense nature of acute wounds the following guidelines provide the ABC of standard procedures: that can help in the various common acute wounds you may see on a day to day basis.

ABRASIONS

Injuries occur in everyday life, and if you're active in sports, you may experience them quite frequently. Almost everyone has experienced an injury called an abrasion. It occurs when skin is rubbed away, like a skinned knee or a road rash. Abrasions can be painful; bleeding starts immediately after the skin is broken. With proper care, minor abrasions heal in a short period of time.

Care

Wash your hands for 15 seconds, then dry them with a clean cloth.

Stop the bleeding by pressing a clean cloth against the wound.

After the bleeding has stopped, rinse the wound with large amounts of cold water.

Do not use iodine solutions, alcohol or soap to clean the abrasion.

Use a clean, damp cloth to gently remove small pieces of dirt.

If bleeding re-occurs after you have cleaned the wound, stop the bleeding again by pressing a clean cloth against the wound.

If you're unable to stop the bleeding in 10 minutes using firm pressure, and/or if there's something in the wound that won't easily rinse out, seek medical attention.

Protect the wound and keep it moist with a non-stick bandage.

For extra protection, use an antibacterial ointment, e.g. bacitracin, polysporin, double antibiotic ointment.

If using neomycin, be aware that it can have allergic effects.

Change the bandage if it gets wet or dirty.

Prevention

It is impossible to prevent all abrasion injuries, but you can decrease the number of abrasion injuries by wearing protective pads and covering exposed skin with a layer of clothing.

BRUISES

A bruise usually occurs after a fall or bump against an object, causing an area of your skin to become purple or dark red in colour from blood that has leaked out of the blood vessels under your skin. The area may at first be swollen and painful; gradually it will become less painful and lighter in colour as your body reabsorbs the blood.

Care

For the first two days after the injury, you may apply cold compresses for 15 to 20 minutes per hour while you're awake, in order to help reduce the pain and swelling.

After 2 days, you may change to warm compresses for 20 minutes per hour while awake for comfort.

Avoid massaging the bruise as this can actually cause more damage.

Caution

Some medical conditions and medications, such as anemia, certain blood diseases, and aspirin or blood thinners, can make a person more prone to bruises. Consult your health care professional about frequent bruising or a bruise that is firm, raised and/or does not begin to fade over a week's time.

CUTS

A cut or laceration is an opening in the skin caused by trauma. It may have straight or jagged edges. Anyone exposed to sharp edges such as knives, screwdrivers, other tools or even paper is at risk of experiencing a skin cut.

Care

Wash and dry your hands.

Apply direct pressure to any bleeding with a clean paper towel or cloth until bleeding has stopped.

Rinse the wound with clean water.

Do not use hydrogen peroxide, iodine solutions, alcohol or soap.

If bleeding continues, reapply pressure. Seek medical help if the bleeding doesn't stop with 10 minutes of firm pressure.

Get a tetanus shot if you're cut by a dirty or rusty object and your shot is not up-to-date.

A topical microbial ointment may be applied over the open area. Again, be alert to possible allergic reactions from neomycin.

Keep the wound clean and moist by placing a clean non-stick bandage over the cut. Keep it covered to prevent scab formation until the skin grows back.

Change the bandage if it becomes wet or soiled.

See your health care professional for a puncture, or jagged or deep cut.

Prevention

Use care whenever you are in a situation where you're exposed to sharp edges.

SKIN TEARS

A skin tear is a separation or peeling back of the outer layer of the skin. It looks like an open blister or loose flap of the skin.

People at risk

Elderly people with fragile skin, wheelchair users, cognitively impaired people and those people needing total care.

Causes of skin tears

Rubbing or sliding the skin.

Removal of tape.

Bumping into furniture or objects.

Falls.

Pulling movements on the arms or legs.

Care practices

Wash your hands for at least 15 seconds.

Gently rinse the wound with clean water.

Pat or air dry the skin.

If there is a loose piece of skin still attached place it back over the wound.

Cover with a non stick, non adhesive pad.

Use gauze wrap or tubular bandage to hold the pad in place.

Do not use tape on the skin.

Change the bandage if it becomes soiled or soaked with drainage; carefully remove the bandage, rinse the wound gently, and apply a new bandage.

Prevention principles

Carefully handle people with fragile skin.

Avoid harsh or pulling movements

Practice extreme care, in keeping with your training, when transferring, turning lifting or positioning patients.

Consider padding side rails, arms or leg supports.

Patients at-risk should wear long sleeves or pants.

Adopt a regular skin care regimen of moisturizing cream or lotion to the skin.

CHRONIC WOUNDS

As the name "chronic" implies, these wounds take a long time to heal and some of these wounds are classified as non – healing or recalcitrant a patient, caregiver or health worker you can have a tremendous impact on the success or failure of the healing process and thereby greatly influence quality of life of the wound sufferer.

Venous, arterial and diabetic ulcers (often referred to as lower extremity ulcers), as well as pressure ulcers, make up the majority of chronic wounds.

Management of these chronic wounds has improved considerably over the past decade as clinicians have realized the importance of proactive measures and a multidisciplinary team approach.

The introduction of newer treatment modalities, such as growth factors and biological skin replacements, holds the promise of treating these difficult wounds, speeding up the wound healing process, and preventing new wound formation.

Early intervention or sustained quality care of a chronic wound is essential: in the fact that 50% of amputations of feet due to diabetic foot ulcers could have been prevented with sustained quality care and patient adherence to treatment.

Without doubt, the biggest concern of chronic ulcers is the effect on quality of life for the patient with regard to a host of parameters such as loss of dignity, embarrassment, social activity, work life and so on. However, chronic ulcers also create the problems go further an enormous workload for health workers, caregivers and health care practitioners, not to mention the enormous financial costs that burden the families, government and insurance companies.

Your constant vigilance, understanding, dialogue, and consistent assessment and documentation of the caring process contribute more to success than any other part of the process.

Recognizing red flags of early warning signs or failure to heal symptoms and being aware of appropriate interventions, can make you the star player of this winning team.

The following overview of the various chronic wounds should provides the foundation of understanding when coupled with the generic information on wound care provided in this book.

The common factor in these chronic wounds is that they take a long time to heal. In all cases it is much better to prevent one of these ulcers forming than trying to heal the ulcer once it has happened.

We have already shown how aging skin contributes to a loss of skin integrity. Such factors as thinning skin, poor blood circulation, risk of infection, and drier skin all contribute to a slow healing, chronic wound.

Therefore, it is important to provide comprehensive care such as good nutrition, optimum skin care, protecting the skin against trauma, and controlling incontinence so that the elderly person has a fighting chance against these challenging situations.

The care of these chronic wounds is the domain of the health care professional involving dressing choices, specific skin care treatments and perhaps special mattresses. There are many other treatment issues that the health provider may have to consider.

You can help in deciding if someone is at-risk for developing one of these skin ulcers and ensure your colleagues are alerted to these at risk patients. For example, a less mobile person is at risk for pressure ulcers, a person with diabetes is at risk for a foot ulcer and people with venous hypertension, demonstrating swelling on the lower legs are at risk for venous leg ulcers.

We must always remember chronic wound care is a team effort involving the patient, caregivers, health workers and the medical staff; each member of the team is equally important in the prevention and healing processes.

Pressure ulcers (bedsores)

This is skin damage due to excess pressure on vulnerable, at risk parts of the skin, mostly around bony prominences like the elbow and heel. Contributing factors putting the patient further at risk include poorly managed incontinence, poor hygiene and an unsafe environment.

The following illustrations depict the areas of the body which are at risk in various situations.

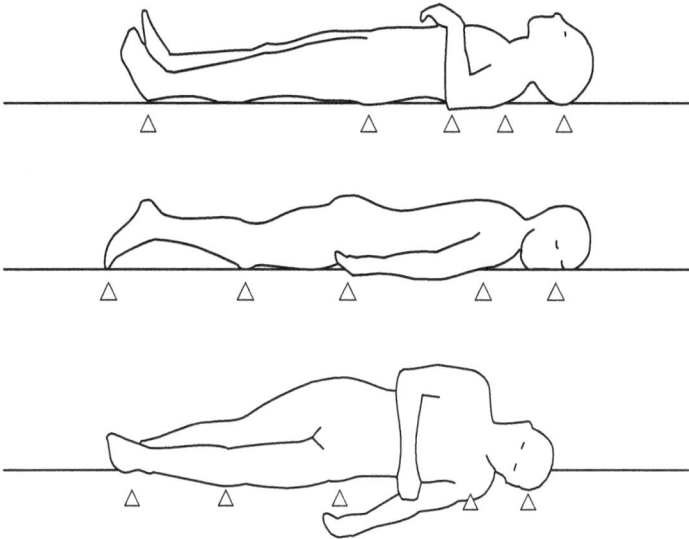

The following illustration shows the at risk areas for shearing and friction forces with a person sliding downwards from the sitting position in bed.

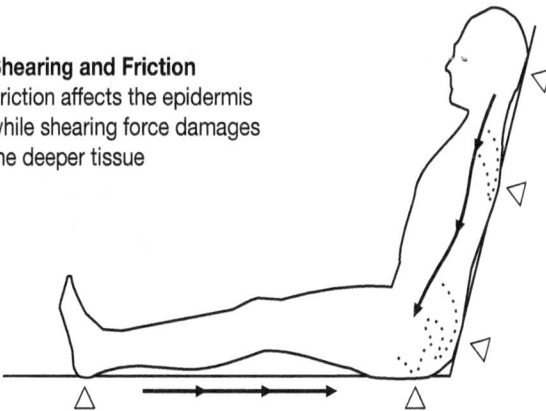

Shearing and Friction
Friction affects the epidermis while shearing force damages the deeper tissue

The stages of a pressure ulcer are shown in the following diagrams as classified by an authoritative body called the NPUAP, the National Pressure Ulcer Advisory Panel.

STAGE I
Description and Symptoms

This is the mild stage, appearing as pink, red, or mottled, unbroken skin that stays that way for more than 20 minutes after the pressure is relieved (an African-American person's skin may look purple.) The skin feels warm and firm (evidence of swelling under the skin.)

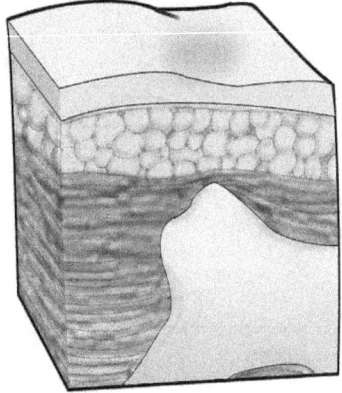

Prognosis
Reversible if you remove the pressure right away.

STAGE II
Description and Symptoms

A blister or a superficial loss of skin appearing as an abrasion or shallow crater. It may be painful and visibly swollen.

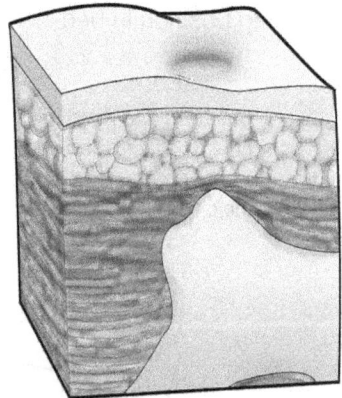

Prognosis
If the pressure is removed, the ulcer can heal in a relatively short time.

STAGE III
Description and Symptoms
A deep crater develops in the skin. Foul-smelling yellow or green fluid may ooze from it if there is infection present. The center is usually not painful because the nerve cells are dead.

Prognosis
It may take months to heal.

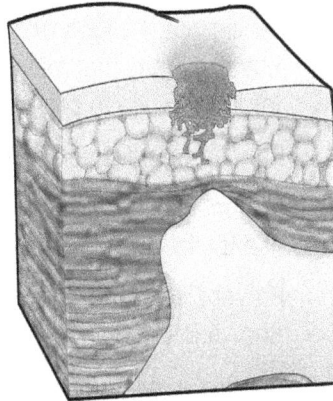

STAGE IV
Description and Symptoms
Tissue is now destroyed from the skin to the bone or close to the bone.

Prognosis
It usually takes a lot of time and costly treatment to heal.

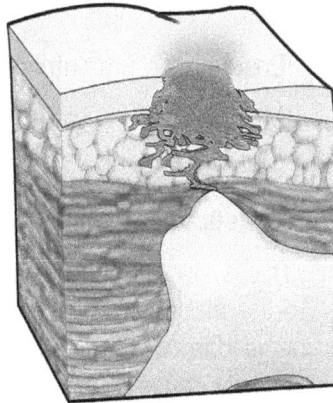

What to do

•For immobile patients ensure turning every two hours, and try to avoid shearing or friction adverse forces.

•Be vigilant, looking at the high risk areas for red spots or hot skin areas that may indicate a pressure ulcer is forming. Inform the health professional immediately.

•Encourage passive/active exercises.

•Protect skin against excess pressure on bony prominences like the heel, elbow and lower back.

•Prevent shearing or friction forces while lying in bed as shown in the diagram.

•Provide a safe environment to avoid a knock or trauma on the skin.

•Manage incontinence through underwear pads and skin care protectant products.

•Avoid excessive perspiration through inappropriate bedding or clothing.

•Ensure optimum nutrition.

•Maintain good hygiene but avoid over - bathing.

Diabetic foot ulcers

This is skin damage on the pressure points on the foot due to the diabetes effect of high blood glucose levels causing nerve damage and blood circulatory problems. These collectively cause a foot to become insensitive or unfeeling so that damage can occur without sensing the damage taking place (like an object lodged in the shoe and pressing on the skin). The poor blood circulation hinders the healing process because vital nutrients have difficulty being carried to the wound site.

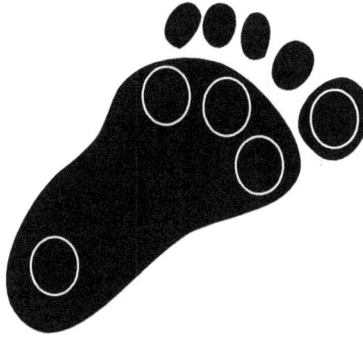

At risk areas of the foot

What to do

- Regular vigilant foot inspections are necessary to check if an ulcer is developing.

- Ensure regular foot care including daily wash and dry, toe-nail care, skin care and lubrication and keep to sensible walking habits.

- Wear recommended protective footwear.

- void pressure on high risk areas of the foot, follow recommendations or wear pressure offloading devices.

- Ensure control of glucose (sugar) levels at all times through the physician's or nurse's recommendations and treatment.

- Encourage recommended lifestyle changes like losing weight or quitting smoking; these can provide enormous benefits.

Venous leg ulcers

This skin damage usually occurs on the lower inside of leg and ankle. The skin damage is due to venous high blood pressure in the capillaries of the skin causing swelling or edema. The damaging result of this swelling is that oxygen and nutrients have difficulty nourishing the skin area and the skin eventually breaks down forming a skin ulcer.

Signs of venous insufficiency

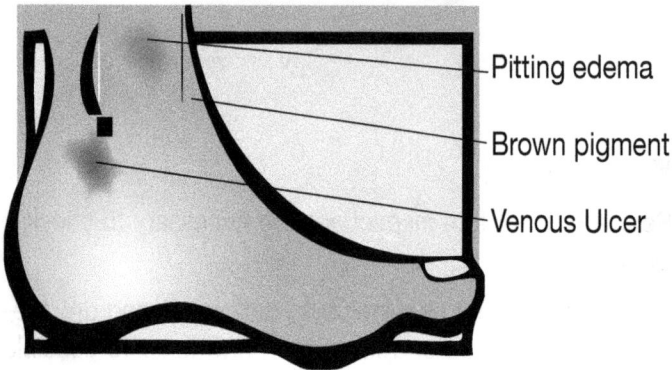

Pitting edema

Brown pigment

Venous Ulcer

What to do

- For symptom relief, encourage the client to keep the legs 6" elevated above the heart by lying on the couch.

- Ensure adherence to using a compression bandage or stocking as recommended by the health care professional

- Help avoid scratching and ensure good hygiene and skin care habits.

•Make sure you ask clients if they are in pain in order to obtain relief.

Arterial ulcers

These are relatively smaller ulcers that can occur on the tips of the toes, heels, nail beds and between the toes, they occur at the farthest end of an arterial branch. They tend to have a "punched out" appearance, are usually black and dry and can be quite painful. The pain can be reduced by lowering the leg. There is no swelling but a sign is a reduced or absent pulse in the area is a possible symptom.

They are caused by poor arterial (oxygeneated) blood flow caused usually by hardening of the arteries (atherosclerosis). Advanced age, smoking, diabetes, high blood pressure and high cholesterol are all risk factors that can contribute to the problem.

What to do

•Be aware that the health professional will assess the comparative arterial blood pressure (called the ABPI, Ankle Brachial Pressure Index) around the ulcer area using a Doppler ultrasound device. This will tell you how bad the arterial blood supply is to the affected area, and determine the prognosis for healing or whether surgery is required.

•Always check for pain and whether medication is needed.

•Pain relief is usually achieved by lowering the foot.

•Inspect the skin regularly for warning signs of a new ulcer, such as an abraded area or skin breakdown.

- Keep to a preventative skin care program with the recommended products.

- Wash the feet daily with mild soap and water and dry carefully between the toes.

- Advise wearing supportive footwear that fits well and recommend not to walk barefoot.

Here's a quick reference distinction between the three types of leg ulcers.

	Venous	Arterial	Diabetic
Location	Inside surface of leg Above the ankle	Top of foot or toes Above or below ankle	Toes Weight bearing surfaces Areas of friction
Shape	Irregular shape Shallow diffuse edge	Punched out appearance Deep "cliff" edge	Punched out Cliff edge/callous
Ulcer Surface Colour	Red / yellow Exuding	Usually black Dry	Often or usually black Dry
Ulcer Size	Medium to large	Small	Small / very small
Edema / Swelling	Generalized lower leg	Localized around ulcer only inflamation	Absent
Leg / Foot Pulses	Normal	Reduced or absent	Present
Pain	Often present Worse with leg down Relieved with leg up	Often present Worse with leg up Relieved with leg down Night pain	Often absent
Skin Staining	Usually	Rarely	Rarely
Ulcer Draining Fluid	Yes	Rarely	Rarely
ABI*	0.8 or above	Below 0.8	Unreliable

NOTES

Pain assessment

You must mention to your physician if you or your client is experiencing a lot of discomfort and pain. While battling wounds you need to be as free from pain as possible to keep up your morale. It is unfortunate that sometimes patients accept the pain as the norm – "it comes with the territory".

Conversely, the onus is with the physician/nurse and also the caregivers and front line health workers to adopt an interventionist policy and ask the right questions to pinpoint the extent of the pain problem.

Painkillers as simple as Ibubrofen, like Motrin can often help or a dressing change can also help relieve pain.

Research has pinpointed many words used by patients to describe their pain: aching, annoying burning, dull, hot, hurting, nagging, sharp, shooting, sick in the stomach pain, stabbing, stinging, throbbing and uncomfortable.

It is important to be aware that the range of pain associated with wounds can vary. Venous and arterial leg ulcers can be very painful, whereas diabetic foot ulcer sufferers do not feel as much pain because of damaged nerves due to diabetes.

Helpful pointers in pain management

a) Use a pain scale tool routinely, involve the patient, and educate the patient on the scale.

b) Pain is subjective, the patient's perception of the pain is the reality. Ask questions to assess nature of the pain and obtain a dialogue.

For example:

- Can you describe the pain?
- What word best describes your pain?
- Where is the pain?
- What makes the pain worse?
- Is the pain worse at night?
- What makes the pain better?
- Are dressing changes painful to you?
- What painkillers are you taking?

c) In order to prevent pain during a debridement or a dressing change it is important to plan and prepare based on your assessment of the patient's pain situation. Here are some suggestions:

- Explain the entire process to the patient.
- Consider preventative analgesia (painkillers).
- Provide a non stressful environment, cell phones turned off, windows closed, quiet setting, etc.
- Avoid prolonged exposure of the ulcer, e.g. waiting for the nurse to arrive.
- Decide if a family member or someone holding hands or touching will help.
- Constantly involve the patient in dialogue to check how they are feeling.
- Make sure the optimum dressing is being used.

NOTES

WOUND CARE PRACTICES

This section is to help you understand all the various procedures that a physician or health care practitioner may perform on a wound. You should never attempt to do the work of a health care practitioner unless you have been requested, instructed and trained to perform the task. We must emphasize that this information is for understanding only and is not intended to provide all the guidelines for a particular wound care activity.

Wound care practices consists of wound assessment, a discipline that attempts to accurately define all the key characteristics and measurements of a wound, and the wound care activities that treat the wound to aid in healing; this involves considerable skills, knowledge, understanding and experience.

WOUND CARE ASSESSMENT

This is the domain of the health care practitioner. After a complete assessment of the patient and the type of wound (diabetic foot ulcer, pressure ulcer etc.), this information is then translated into specific treatment requirements.

There are other specific assessments made for a particular type of wound. For example, there are four "staging" category assessments for pressure ulcers and a blood flow measurement test called the ABPI for venous leg ulcer patients. .

If you are called upon to do some assessing you should remember that it does not matter what methods you use to record your observations as long as you are consistent.

Measuring the wound

In order to assess progress in the healing of a wound it is important to regularly measure a wound. The length, width and depth should be noted but also the skin surrounding the skin should be described and defined.

Measuring the length – you should determine the longest distance across the open area of the wound, regardless of the shape of the wound.

Measuring the width – next you should determine the longest distance at a right angle to the axis of the length measurement.

Classifying wound depth

A wound is normally classified as partial thickness or full thickness according to its depth.

Partial thickness wounds involve only the epidermis; they extend into the dermis but not through it.

These wound usually heal quickly because they involve only the epidermal layer of the skin. They are also less susceptible to infection because part of the body's first line of defense (partial dermis) is still intact.

Full thickness wounds extend through the dermis into tissues beneath and may expose adipose tissue, muscle or even bone. These wounds require more body resources and more time to heal than partial thickness wounds. When assessing a full thickness wound, the depth should be reported as well as the length and width.

Measuring the depth of a wound.

To measure wound depth, wear a pair of gloves and then gently insert a flexible foam-tipped device into the deepest portion of the wound. Carefully mark the stick where it meets the edge of the skin. Remove the device and measure the distance from your mark to the end, to determine the depth.

Measuring tunneling and undermining

It is also important to measure and obtain the direction of tunnels, or extensions of the wound bed into adjacent tissue.

You measure tunnels and undermining just as you would wound depth with the exception that you insert the applicator where the tunneling occurs. See the illustration.

View the direction of the applicator as if it were the hand of a clock where 12 o'clock points in the direction of the patient's head.

Progressing in a clockwise direction, document the deepest site where the wound actually tunnels—for example "three o'clock."

Assessing drainage

This is a critical issue because incorrect management of the wound exudates can cause further problems.

To properly assess drainage you should observe the dressing before you remove it and answer the following questions so that you can obtain a thorough understanding of the situation:

- If the dressing is occlusive were the dressing edges well sealed?
- Does the drainage ooze from the edges of the dressing?
- Is there an odour coming from the dressing?
- Is the dressing saturated or dry?
- How much drainage is there—scant, moderate or a large amount?
- How would you describe the drainage with regard to consistency, texture and colour?

Description of the Drainage

Description	Colour and consistency
Serous	Clear or light yellow Thin and watery
Sanguineous	Red (traces of blood) Thin
Serosanguineous	Pink to light red Thin and watery
Purulent	Creamy yellow, tan, green or white Thick and opaque

Wound colour clues classification

The red – yellow – black classification system is a commonly used approach that can help you determine how well the wound is healing. If you observe more than one colour in the wound, classify it according to the least healthy colour.

Reddened	Red	Yellow	Black
Warning	More healthy	Less healthy	Least healthy

Pre-ulcerative (reddened skin) phase

In this phase there is usually no break in the skin; however, there are ominous signs of reddening and sometimes swelling and being warm to the touch. Unless appropriate basic intervention steps are taken, imminent tissue breakdown is a possibility. This phase is the most easily reversible through sensible intervention, perhaps by removing the source of pressure or friction/shearing and protecting the tissue from excessive moisture and further trauma. Improving the blood supply to the area could also help. Basic skin care is pivotal to the success of treatment using cleansers, moisturizers and/or protective creams and ointments.

Choice of dressing

The key issues are to protect the skin at all costs; to prevent further trauma. One should be able to remove the dressing without damaging the skin. The nature of the dressing should not encourage the "softening" (macerating) of both healthy and "at-risk" skin but should support a healthy skin environment.

Granulation (red) phase

This dominant red appearance is evidence of a clean wound which is either ready to heal or is actually healing. The dominant theme of this phase is the obvious regenerative nature of the wound – new cell growth. Only superficial tissue loss is apparent with skin loss occurring only in the epidermis or dermis. The wound could look like an abrasion, blister or shallow crater. This type of wound appears clean with a pink or red base or clusters of growing tissue. The drainage from the wound may be simply a thin, watery fluid (serous) or mixed with blood (serosanguinous).

Damage can occur to the subcutaneous tissue, showing itself as quite a deep crater. Again, because of the granulating or rapid healing process of skin growth, the wound appears clean with a pink to red bed or small granulating clusters. This time the serous or serosanguinous drainage may be not mild but heavy.

Choice of dressing

In this active stage, dressings serve many purposes. Let's review the various factors:

- Maintaining a clean and moist environment. This is vital for cell growth and migration necessary for healing. The maintenance of a moist wound surface prevents wound desiccation (drying up) which is detrimental to the healing process.

- Absorbing excess exudates: Too much wound exudate can soften (macerate) surrounding tissues. In fact, large amounts of wound exudate can dilute wound healing factors and nutrients at the wound surface. Also, the toxins made by bacteria in the wound can further inhibit the wound repair process so the dressing should absorb these toxins to optimize the healing process.

•Protect newly-formed tissue. Obviously, any infection or trauma to the healing wound can delay recovery so it is very important that the dressing not stick to the wound surface and also protect the wound from the outside.

•Maintain a thermally-insulated wound environment. Keeping normal tissue temperature improves blood flow to the wound bed and helps in cell migration.

•Obliterate "dead space". By dead space, we mean the areas of empty space between the skin surface and wound floor, underlying intact surface tissues.

Clearly, there are dressings that fulfill these criteria and should be used as instructed by the manufacturer. Aggressive treatment at this phase can halt the progression to the inflammation and necrotic phases which are more difficult to treat. Site management usually involves cleaning the wound with saline solution.

Inflammatory (yellow) phase

This is a highly active phase with an obvious yellow fibrous debris or thick surface exudate present. Granulation tissue maybe visible but the major concern here is looking for signs of infection. Wound drainage will be moderate to heavy and pus may be present.

Inflammation and infection can delay the healing process so

the choice of dressing is critical. Again, site management will call for cleansing the wound with saline but debris will also have to be removed, either mechanically or with assistance from an appropriate wound product.

Choice of dressing

There are many dressing options, again this is the decision of the health care professional. :

- •Supporting the natural cleansing mechanism of the wound. Keeping the wound clean is vital to ensure there is no further exacerbation of infection.

- •Absorbing excess exudate. Too much exudate can soften (macerate) the surrounding skin and make it vulnerable. Dilution of wound healing factors and nutrients can slow down the healing process. It is important that in this phase a dressing be able to absorb bacterial toxins.

- •Supporting the removal of necrotic (dead) or foreign tissue from the wound. This can prevent further inflammation.

- •Discouraging bacterial growth. This will help to reduce infection.

Necrotic (black) phase

The wound may now be partially or completely covered with black eschar (dry crust) or with loose or string-like necrotic tissue, which may be black, brown or gray in colour. There may be purulent (pus-like) or fibrous material at the edges of the wound.

This black phase is usually quite advanced and considerable site management is necessary. Besides the usual cleansing with saline, it is vital to remove the debris (debridement) of necrotic tissue.

Dead tissue can cause further inflammation and/or provide an environment for bacterial growth, as well as slowing down the healing process. It is up to the medical team to decide how this tissue should be debrided from the wound.

Choice of dressing

There are many options for this category. Obviously, it is very important to choose a dressing that provides effective debridement as well as minimizing the risk of infection. Only health care professionals can make the decision for this situation because there are other variables; a wound with an inadequate blood supply for instance may just need to be kept clean and dry.

Skin colour markers

The colour of the skin around the wound can be a "red flag" to future problems that can hinder the healing process.

White skin indicates maceration, a result of too much moisture and suggests the need for a protective barrier around the wound and possibly a more absorbent dressing.

Red skin can indicate inflammation, injury e.g. a tape burn or pressure, or infection. It is important to find out the cause of this inflammation.

Purple skin can indicate bruising, a sign of perhaps an inappropriate environment, such as furniture clutter.

SIGNS & CAUSES OF FAILURE TO HEAL

This succinct chart pinpoints what you should be looking for to determine if there is a problem with a wound healing. In form the health care professional and for your information the various interventions are outlined

SIGNS	CAUSES	INTERVENTIONS
WOUND EDGES		
Red , hot, tender	Excess pressure Infection	Protect area from pressure Antimicrobial therapy
Maceration, soft white skin	Incontinence Excess moisture	Underpads, or skin protectant Use absorptive dressing
Rolled skin edges	Too dry wound bed	Moisture retentive dressing Possible debridement on the edges
Undermining or loose Bruised skin edges	Shearing forces	Protect the area especially during patient transfers.

SIGNS	CAUSES	INTERVENTIONS
WOUND BED		
Too dry	Exposure of tissue to air. Inadequate hydration	Add moisture on a regular basis. Use a dressing that maintains moisture
Increase in size or depth	Infection Result of debridement Local pressure Check any of the factors that retard healing	If caused by debridement no intervention necessary. Comprehensive reassessment of the patient.
Increase in size or depth	Poor circulation or a pressure point Infection	Medical intervention necessary
Necrosis	Poor circulation (ischemia)	Carry out debridement if there is adequate circulation.
Negative change in drainage	Infection Type of debridement	Reassess the wound
Tunneling Pressure point	Presence of foreign body Deep infection	Protect area from pressure. Inspect and irrigate tunnel. Obtain biopsy for infection or malignancy.

Complications of wound healing

You may come across some complications of wound healing which are important to be aware of in order to realize immediate medical is necessary.

Infection

This condition requires immediate attention because, if left untreated, bacterial infection or cellulites could develop and spread to surrounding tissues. Here are the signs and symptoms to look out for:

- Fever
- Edema (swelling)
- Pain at the wound site or sudden increase in existing pain
- Pus exuding
- A distinct odour
- Redness or warmth at the wound margins and the surrounding tissue
- Discloured granulation tissue
- An increase in the exudates or drainage or a change in its colour
- More wound (breakdown) or lack of progress towards healing

Hemorrhage (bleeding)

Bleeding from the wound can result from the rupture of newly developed blood capillaries. Each time the new blood capillary suffers damage, the body has to repair the capillaries which further delays healing. This factor provides another good reason to protect the wound with a dressing.

Fistula formation

A fistula is an abnormal passage between two organs or between an organ and skin. This may appear as a tunnel or undermining and it is important to both measure and determine the direction in order to monitor progress.

Dehiscence and evisceration

This phenomenon can be serious. Dehiscence is a separation of the skin and tissue layers. It usually occurs 3 to 12 days after the injury or after surgery.

Evisceration is more specifically the protrusion of an underlying visceral organ such as the bowel.

Both these conditions may require emergency surgery, especially if they involve an abdominal wound. Conversely, if a wound opens without evisceration, it may heal by the secondary intention manner of healing.

Advanced age and poor nutrition can increase the risk of these two problems.

NOTES

WOUND CARE ACTIVITIES

The wound care plan

Nature is the most powerful ally in wound healing and the most sound and simple approach to wound healing is to keep the wound moist, free of debris and well protected. However there will be specific requirements based on the nature of the chronic wound and the assessment of the patient requiring the development of an individual wound care plan for each patient.

The wound care plan should include the following:

•Provide nutritional and fluid support.

•Establish and maintain a clean, moist, protected wound bed.

•Ensure optimum management of wound exudates and drainage.

•Remove dead tissue (debridement) as needed.

•Protect the integrity of the skin surrounding the wound, ensuring it stays dry and intact.

•Try to improve blood supply to the wound.

•Prevent or effectively manage infection as quickly as possible.

This wound care plan is by nature a dynamic plan where constant reassessment can shift priorities. For example, if the wound does not change within two weeks, you will have to reassess the patient's condition and wound, look for negative factors slowing the healing process and revise the plan. If there is no apparent healing after a period of four weeks of treatment, a wound care specialist should evaluate the situation.

Wound plan decision making checklist

After all the assessment has taken place, the health care professional needs to address the following questions, related to the wound care plan. This can be helpful in understanding the planning process. The planning process is of course dependant upon the facility's policies, procedures and product formulary.

- Has there been a comprehensive wound assessment completed?
- Is the wound clean or necrotic?
- Is debridement necessary?
- How should the wound be cleaned?
- Is the wound infected?
- Is there an opportunity to prevent new wounds forming?
- How much drainage is currently present?
- Is the skin surrounding the wound healthy?
- Is the blood flow to the wound adequate?
- Has the pain issue been addressed?
- What dressing is appropriate?
- How will the patient/caregiver be educated and involved?

CHOICE OF DRESSING

Your medical team will provide a dressing designed to meet the specific needs of your wound. There is no one dressing available that can provide a perfect environment for all wounds. Most clinicians, with this in mind, have an arsenal of dressings, so they can choose the right dressing for the right patient at the right time. Try to be an informed consumer with regard to dressings because the clinician will find your comments helpful when it comes to the following matters:

•Any pain you may experience during dressing changes.

•Any discomfort.

•Whether you find any odors from the wound offensive or perhaps offensive to family members. Always tell the clinician about any odors from the wound because it could mean a change of dressing is necessary to fight infection.

•Is there risk from damaging the wound? If so, protection may be required.

•Do you and the clinician agree on how many times the dressing should be changed and the length of time it will take to heal?

Here are the various categories of dressings with some common brand names included. This classification is not a rigid one as there are many hybrid or composite dressings that combine aspects of members of different groups in order to achieve an optimum effect:

Transparent films

These are polyurethane based and transparent with varying thickness and adhesive coatings on one side only (to adhere to the skin). These dressings are impermeable to bacteria and fungi but can be permeated by moisture and oxygen. Brand names: Sure Site™, Tegaderm™, Carrafilm™, Comfeel®, Bioclusive*, Transeal®, Polyskin® and OpSite*.

Gauzes and non-woven dressings

These are available as sponges or wraps and, depending on their design, have varying degrees of absorbency. They are made of cotton, rayon or polyester and are available as sterile or non-sterile.

Brand names: Curity Gauze Sponges, Carrington® Bordered Gauze, Avant Gauze™, CovRSite® Cover, Telfar, FLUFTEX™and Medline® Bordered Gauze.

Soft silicone mesh

This is a non-adhering, porous, semi-transparent dressing with a wound contact layer consisting of flexible polyamide net coated with soft silicone. Although it is nonabsorbent, the porous nature allows fluid to pass through to the secondary dressing. Primarily used in skin donor sites. Brand name: Mepitel®.

Hydrocolloids

These are composed of carboxymethylcellulose (a sort of heavy carbohydrate), gelatin or pectin and have different absorption capabilities depending upon their thickness and composition. They are waterproof, impermeable to bacteria, promote autolytic debridement and can be changed every 3 to 7 days. Absorption, however, is limited. These are useful in granulating and epithializing wounds with minimal exudates. Brand names: Duo Derm®, Comfeel® Plus, 3M™ Tegasorb™, CaraColloid™, Procol®, Permacol™, Restore™, NU-DERM* BORDER, AquaTack™, ExuDERM™, CUTINOVA* Hydro, RepliCare® and Ultec®.

Alginates

These are non-woven sheets or ropes composed of natural polysaccharide fibers derived from seaweed. They are comfortable and good for heavy exuding wounds. However, they may cause drying of the wound if it is not producing enough fluid. Brand names: Kaltostat®, Curasorb®, Sorbsan®, 3M™ Tegagen™, SeaSorb® Soft, CarraGinate™, NU-DERM*, Maxorb™ Melgisorb®, AlgiSite*, and CURASORB®.

Biologicals and biosynthetics

These are gels, solutions or semi-occlusive sheets derived from a natural source. They act as sort of scaffolds to promote healing of the tissues. Brand names: Oasis®, BIOBRANE® and Apilagraf®.

Collagen dressings

These can be particles, sheets, and amorphous dressings; as the name implies, collagen is derived from animal sources. These dressings encourage the deposition and organization of newly formed collagen fibers and granulation tissue within the wound bed. Brand names: FIBRACOL* and PRO-MOGRAN* and Woun'Dres®.

Cavity fillers

As the name suggests these dressings fill in dead space within the wound and can be in the form of beads, foam, gel, pillow, strand, ointment or paste. Their function is to keep the wound moist and absorb exudates. A secondary dressing for protection is required over the cavity filler. Brand names: Flex-igel® Strands®, Carrasorb™, TRIAD™ and MULTIDEX®.

Absorptives

These are multilayered wound cover dressings that provide either a semi-adherent quality or non-adherent layer, combined with highly absorptive layers of fiber, such as cotton, rayon or cellulose. They are designed to minimize wound trauma and manage moderate exudates. Brand names: Mepore®, Covaderm®, Aquacel®, Primapore*, IODOFLEX™, SOFSORB®.

Contact layers

These are thin sheets of non-adherent material placed in the wound bed to protect granulating tissue from other potentially destructive dressings. These dressings conform to the shape of the wound bed and, being porous, allow wound fluids and exudates to flow through for absorption by a secondary dressing. Brand names: Mepitel®, 3M™ Tegapore™, Profore* and DERMANET®.

Foams

These are absorptive sheets and shapes of formed polymer solutions such as polyurethane, with small open cells, which hold fluids and have non-adherent layers. They are easy to apply and remove and are useful with wounds with large volumes of exudates. Some foam dressings are available in both non-adhesive and adhesive versions, which do not require a secondary dressing.

Brand names: Allevyn*, Optifoam™, PolyMem®, 3M™ Foam Adhesive, Lyofoam®, POLYDERM™, Hydrofera Blue™, SOF-FOAM*, TIELLE*, Mepilex®, CURAFOAM® and Biatain™. Other foams are available that secure the dressing in place during application while minimizing trauma to granulation tissue on removal. Brand name: Biatain Soft-Hold.

Hydrogel dressings

These are primarily composed of water and are designed to donate moisture to the wound site. Some special formula actually absorb exudates as well – a "smart" dressing. Brand names: Intrasite*, TenderWet®, SkinTegrity™ Hydrogel, 3M™ Tegagel™, Carrasmart™, Purilon™, DuoDERM®, Dermagran®, CURASOL®, NU- GEL*, IntraSite* and SoloSite®.

Impregnated dressings

These include gauzes and non-woven sponges, ropes and strips that are saturated with a solution, emulsion, oil agent or compound including saline, petroleum, zeroform, zinc salts, iodine or scarlet red. Brand names: Vaseline Petrolatum Gauze®, Adaptic* Non Adhering Dressing.

Active Dressings

1)Silver dressings

These deliver a sustained release, broad spectrum, anti-microbial action while maintaining a moist environment for the wound. Available as many different dressing types, their objective is to treat or reduce the risk of infection. Brand names: Acticoat*, Arglaes®, SilvaSorb™ and Contreet®.

2) Pain relief

The only available brand, Biatain-Ibu, is a foam dressing with a built-in analgesic, Ibuprofen, which is delivered directly to the wound site, and thereby may relieve both temporary pain (during dressing change) and persistent pain, as well as manage the wound exudate.

Composites

These are wound covers that possess more than one component to address the multiple wound care needs and dressing functions. They can function as primary or secondary dressings.

Brand names: Telfa® Plus Barrier Island, 3M™ Tegaderm™, Plus Pad Transparent dressing with absorbent pad, 3M™ Medipore™, COVADERMPLUS®, CovRSite® and TELFA®.

All these dressings try to address the major goals of providing cover, protection, hydration (keeping moist), insulation and absorption, as well as preventing infection, filling dead space, promoting granulation (healing) and debridement. Each category of dressing fits some or most of these needs; deciding which to use requires the skill and judgement of a health care practitioner.

The Agency for Health Care Policy and Research (AHCPR), which is an authoritative clinical body, has made critical dressing recommendations, the most important of which are as follows:

•A dressing should keep the ulcer bed moist. Healing has been found to be faster when the wound bed is kept moist.

•The skin surrounding the ulcer should be kept dry. This is to prevent the surrounding skin from becoming damaged.

•A dressing, although absorbing exudates, should not dry out or desiccate the wound bed.

NOTES

CHANGING A DRESSING

Wounds go through stages of healing. The physician or nurse will vary the selection, size and frequency of dressing change according to the type of wound. The following guidelines are for basic dressing change and cleaning procedures:

•Put on gloves.

•Remove all hand jewelry.

•Wash your hands thoroughly before handling the gloves.

•When you have both gloves on, check to be sure there are no breaks in the glove material. If you find any, discard the gloves and start again with a new set.

Applying a gauze dressing

If the person you're caring for has a draining bedsore, you'll need to change the dressing regularly. Begin by assembling your equipment: dressings (regular gauze or nonstick gauze pads), scissors, adhesive tape, cleaning solution prescribed by the doctor, baby oil and a plastic disposal bag. Have the new dressing ready before removing the old one. Cut strips of adhesive tape in advance.

Before you start, position the person so you can easily reach the wound site.

Tip: If the doctor prescribes medication to make dressing changes less painful, give the medication to the patient 1/2 hour before changing the dressing.

Removing the old dressing

Wash your hands thoroughly.

Remove the tape carefully from the patient's skin, leaving

the old dressing in place for now. If necessary to make removal less painful, moisten the old tape with baby oil before you remove it. If the skin under the old tape is inflamed, don't apply the new tape there.

Remove the old dressing, but don't touch any part of it that touched the ulcer. Fold together the edges of the dressing, place it in the disposal bag and close the bag tightly.

Checking the ulcer

Check for swelling, redness, drainage, pus, all of which are signs of probable infection. Is the wound healing? Check the amount and color of drainage on the old dressing. Do not touch the ulcer.

Whether the ulcer appears to be infected, healing or unchanged since the last dressing change, write down what you see; do this every time you change the dressing.

WOUND BED PREPARATION (DEBRIDEMENT)

This is vital aspect of treatment designed to accelerate healing by way of preventing barriers to healing and enhancing the effectiveness of other therapeutic measures. Debridement is considered the order of the day for achieving an optimum wound bed healing surface. Debridement treatment is the activity of removing the dead tissue on top of the wound known as the crust, scab or eschar, or simply blood clots. There are four methods of accomplishing this:

a) Surgical, where the dead tissue is removed by a scalpel or scissors;

b) Mechanical, using a range of techniques including wet-to-dry dressings, wound irrigation or whirlpool soaks;

c) Enzymatic, using various substances to biochemically clear away debris. These products are notavailable in Canada but are available in the US.

d) Autolytic, where certain dressings like hydrogels enhance the effectiveness of the body's own enzymes in debriding dead tissue.

Three further actions of wound bed preparation include:

•Reducing bacteria burden by using topical antiseptics delivered through silver-based dressings or cadexomer iodine.

*Correcting underlying cases of poor circulation and immuno -suppression may also help.

•Maintaining moisture balance, which involves the control of exudate while maintaining a moist wound environment.

This is achieved through the correct use of hydrogel or absorbent dressings or through the use of mechanical devices such as topical negative pressure therapy.

Cleaning a wound

The reasons for cleaning a wound are to remove bacteria and debris from the wound surface and surrounding area. You should always clean a wound before applying a new dressing.

This procedure should focus on the patient's comfort needs and a constructive caring dialogue to allay patient fears and encourage cooperation during the procedure.

The patient should be positioned to maximize his comfort while allowing easy access to the wound site.

Bed linens should be covered with a liner – saver pad to prevent soiling.

Although the health care practitioner should perform this activity, it is worth being familiar with all the items involved in the procedure as listed depending on the facility's policies and resources):

Hypoallergenic tape	Overbed table
Piston – type irrigating system	Recommended cleaning solution
Scissors	Clean or sterile bowl
Sterile 4'x 4" gauze pads	Topical dressing
Impervious trash bag	Disposable wound measuring device
Two pairs of clean sterile gloves	Sterile cotton – tipped applicators

Irrigating a wound

Irrigating a wound cleans tissues and flushes cell debris and exudates from an open wound; it also prevents the formation of a premature surface over an infected tract or an abscess.

This procedure is carried out by a health care practitioner and the items used in irrigation procedures are the same as those listed in the wound cleaning procedure with the addition of:

Emesis basin	Protective eyewear
Gown	Soft rubber or plastic catheter
Clean or sterile container	Sterile irrigation and dressing set
Skin protectant wipe	Prescribed irrigant, such as sterile or non–sterile normal saline solution or sterile water

The equipment should be assembled conveniently in the patient's room. Check the equipment for expiry dates on the sterile packages and for tears.

Any solution that has been opened for 24 hours should not be used; and the solutions used should be at room temperature or warmed to 90° - 95° F.

The trash bag should be opened and placed near the patient's bed, form a cuff by turning down the top of the trash bag.

Pulsatile lavage

This is a new procedure for wound debridement. A wand like device is held close to the wound tissue surface and delivers a sterile irrigating solution under pressure. Concurrent suction is also applied.

A variety of equipment is needed such as needle and syringe combinations, pressurized canisters or battery–powered disposable irrigation systems.

An analgesic is usually administered 20 minutes before the procedure or an I.V. analgesic may be administered immediately before the procedure.

It is important to explain the procedure to the patient and make sure she is relaxed as well as ensure privacy.

The pressure and suction intensity varies according to the nature of the wound as shown:

Wound type

Clean or granulating .... Low pressure/suction

Infected...................................... higher pressure/suction

Necrotic .... Highest pressure/suction

Wet to Dry Dressing procedure

This sterile procedure is typically used for wounds with extensive necrotic tissue and minimal drainage.

Once again explain the procedure to the patient and try to ensure the patient is relaxed and privacy is assured.

The use of an analgesic 20 minutes before the procedure will be necessary.

WARMING (THERAPEUTIC HEAT)

Traditionally, the primary objective of the application of warmth to wounds had been to relieve pain. Preoperative warming is now a standard anesthetic practice.

However, there appear to be other benefits, such as improving blood flow and oxygen tension in tissues, and reducing the risk of developing chronic wounds and decreasing the rate of wound infection in surgery. It may also eradicate certain infections in wounds.

Warming may be applied systemically or locally.

Systemic warming is usually done with specialized warming blankets

Local warming is achieved by specially designed pads that may use an external source of electricity.

Warming is an attractive option for many reasons. It can be used prophylact as well as therapeutically, it is simple to apply, it's inexpensive and cost effective, it may reduce the need for antibiotics and it may actually be useful in circumstances where antibiotics have failed.

NEGATIVE PRESSURE WOUND THERAPY (NPWT)

This innovative and well proven system / device uses negative pressure on a wound to help promote healing through multiple mechanisms of action. The product is classified as a standard dressing treatment option as it has been proven so effective in helping wound healing.

ELECTRICAL STIMULATION

This is the use of an electrical current to transfer energy to a chronic wound. There are many different waveforms available on electrotherapy equipment; the most favorable one for clinical application is HVPC (High Voltage Pulsed Current), which has been proven to be safe and effective.

Used by physical therapists for spasms and injuries, there is increasing interest in this treatment to speed up closure of chronic wounds. In one clinical study it was found that there was significant improvement in patients receiving TENS (transcutaneous electrical nerve stimulators) treatment for skin ulcers compared to patients who used a placebo (a false TENS treatment).

In its clinical practice guidelines, the AHRQ recommends considering electrotherapy treatment for certain stages of pressure ulcers.

The treatment is believed to increase blood flow, enhance tissue oxygenation, reduce edema, control infection, dissolve blood products including necrotic tissue, and stimulate the biochemical rebuilding process.

HYPERBARIC OXYGEN

Oxygen is more than a nutrient. Most vital cellular and molecular repair processes within a chronic wound are directly or indirectly influenced by the available levels of oxygen. This is seen in the poor healing rates among patients with poor blood circulation and the improvement in healing when warming treatment increases the levels of tissue oxygen.

Hyperbaric oxygen is one proven method of increasing oxygen delivery to the tissues. It is achieved by patients breathing in 100% oxygen in pressurized chambers.

The best way of describing how this works is to consider the process of trying to dissolve salt. When you pour a spoonful of salt into a glass of cold water, not all of the salt dissolves. Pour the same amount of salt into hot water and all the salt dissolves. What higher temperatures do for salt in water, pressure does for oxygen in the blood.

The process involves walking into a chamber, alone or with one or more people, while you breathe oxygen through a mask or head tent. Alternatively, you may lie in a one-person chamber, the entire chamber being pressurized and filled with oxygen. It is the oxygen you breathe in, not the circulating oxygen drifting around your pressure ulcer or wound, that helps speed up healing.

For several hours after a treatment, oxygen levels remain high, encouraging capillary growth. New capillaries mean more blood gets to the site of the pressure ulcer, which can speed up healing. This treatment should be regarded as just part of the treatment process; dressings, nutrition, infection control and other aspects of treatment should also be carried out in order for healing to take place.

SKIN SUBSTITUTES

That "skin is the best dressing" is a well-known medical aphorism. The normal structural and cellular components of skin not only have a barrier function on the wound or pressure ulcer but also exert an active, positive influence on the wound environment.

Tissue engineering has provided us with a number of clinically viable options to graft skin onto a wound or pressure ulcer. These products may be single layered (containing the equivalent of either epidermis or dermis) or bilayered (containing layers which mimic both the dermis and epidermis).

GROWTH FACTORS

Normal wound healing is heavily dependent on a wide range of growth factors and cytokines which interact with cells and the matrix at different phases. Topical (applied to the skin) use of growth factors to speed up wound healing.

Maggot Debridement Therapy (MDT)

Repulsive as it may sound, this treatment has proven to be effective with pressure ulcers with slough and infection and can be useful against drug resistant strains of bacteria, such as Methicillin Resistant Staphylococcus Aureus, or MRSA.

Larva therapy involves the application onto the wound of necrophagous larvae of the green bottle fly (Lucilia sericata), reared in a controlled and sterile environment.

Larva therapy is cost-effective and well-tolerated. Maggots augment wound healing in the following ways:

•Having an antimicrobial effect;

•Selective debridement: secreted proteases cause rapid and selective degradation of dead tissue

•Larval secretions promote constructive tissue interactions at the wound site.

The limitations of this treatment are the lack of esthetic appeal and the short life of the maggots.

CONCLUSION: prevention versus treatment.

In the introduction we emphasized it is much better to prevent a wound from occurring than to have to treat a wound. Treating a wound can take a lot of time, care - giving and expense.

Perhaps the most important information contained in this book are the listed early signs and symptoms of a potential wounds forming, such as a tender warm red spot, prior to a pressure ulcer developing or swelling and brown spots around the ankle prior to a venous leg ulcer developing.

Vigilance and consistency in inspecting skin together with an understanding of wound development can help your patient or family member; or if you are a health worker, can help your facility or institution maintain high quality care standards.

Traditionally in health care, expertise has been recognized by finding a cure or intervening in a crisis situation. It has always been an intangible to recognize good quality preventative care of patients and thereby preventing health problems, because health data usually only recognizes quantitative diagnosed health problems.

All this is changing now, and there is positive acknowledgement of good preventative quality care with people at risk for chronic wounds by way of accredited quality care standards with relevant inspection and audits of facilities and institutions.

Prevention is the order of the day for wound care, not only for preventing a wound developing but also as an integral part of the treatment. It is recommended that for the obvious benefit of patients and maintaining high standards within an institution or facility, health workers, caregivers and family members of patients should adopt a preventative focus to caring so that constructive self care habits and quality care procedures always address these principles front and centre.

Review the following chart to reinforce the importance of prevention in your day to day activities.

Prevention Versus Treatment

Prevention Method	Treatment Method
Little effort needed.	Demanding for both patient and caregiver.
Patient comfort assured.	Possible patient stress, discomfort and pain.
Patient in control.	Patient dependent upon medical staff.
Not expensive.	Costly due to medications, dressings, laundry, medical staff, etc.
Medical staff less involved— perhaps in advisory capacity.	Medical staff actively involved.
No presciptions necessary.	Prescibed medications sometimes needed.
Safe procedures.	Risk of complications.
Reduces hospital stay.	Can increase time of hospitalization.
Post hospitalization seldom required.	Continued post hospitalization services, medical appointments necessary.
No recurrence possible.	Recurrence possible.

USEFUL WEBSITES

Canadian Association of Wound Care *see page 84
www.cawc.net

Canadian Association of Enterostomal Therapy
www.caet.ca

Registered Nurses Association of Ontario *see page 84
www.rnao.org

Wound Ostomy & Continence Nurses Association
www.wocn.org

National Pressure Ulcer Advisory Panel *see page 84
www.npuap.org

The Wound Healing Society
www.woundheal.org

American Academy of Wound Management
www.aawm.org

Pressure Ulcer Awareness Program
www.preventpressureulcers.com

International Wound Care Course (IIWC)
www.twhc.ca

Body1.inc
www.wounds1.com

The Wound Care information network
www.medicedu.com

Association for the advancement of wound care
www.aawc1.com

Wound Care Institute
www.woundcare.org

World Wide Wounds
www.worldwidewounds.com

European Pressure Ulcer Advisory Panel
www.epuap.org